PREVENTION IS THE CURE FOR CANCER

PREVENTION IS THE CURE FOR CANCER

5 Easy Steps

TRUDY PIEPER, ND

WESTBOW°
PRESS
A DIVISION OF THOMAS NELSON
& ZONDERVAN

WestBow Press books may be ordered through booksellers or by contacting:

WestBow Press
A Division of Thomas Nelson & Zondervan
1663 Liberty Drive
Bloomington, IN 47403
www.westbowpress.com
1 (866) 928-1240

ISBN: 978-1-4908-7585-9 (sc)
ISBN: 978-1-4908-7584-2 (e)

Library of Congress Control Number: 2015905488

Print information available on the last page.

WestBow Press rev. date: 04/16/2015

To my sisters, Judy Dee and Jody, and sister-in-law, Rose, who have always encouraged me to enjoy life to the fullest. Sisters are a precious gift from God. Their ever-present love and support has helped me to find balance in my life. Through the decades, our bond has continued to grow, and I value them more each day.

Contents

Acknowledgment

I am grateful to my husband, Hal, for not only his loving support for over forty years, but for his research skills and can-do spirit. This book would have never been possible without his aid and assistance. And to my children, Ben, Ken, and Christina, who have always been my inspiration to find a better way to dynamic health.

To the many people who have allowed me the privilege of providing a guide to improve their health, I offer a heart-felt thank you. Without your health issues, I would never have been able to become a super sleuth for health—something I love to do!

Preface

> Lord, make me an instrument of your peace. Where there is hatred, let me sow love. Where there is darkness, let me bring light. Where there is sadness, let me bring joy.
>
> —Prayer of Saint Francis of Assisi

This book is about prevention. However, know that if you already have disease in your body, you can step out in faith and God will meet you. The story of the ten lepers in Luke 17 is a vivid picture of God asking man to join him in a miracle. You know the story. Ten men were hanging out on the back side of the crowd as Christ came through their town, their limbs wrapped in dirty linens. As the law of the day demanded, they limped along at a respectful distance from the crowd, hoping to catch Christ's attention. And unlike most of the healings in the Bible, once in Christ's sights, the men were told to report to the priests to be healed. Jesus wanted them to personally experience faith. Hebrews 11:1 tells us, "Faith is the assurance of things hoped for, the conviction of things not seen."

When the only leper returned to thank Christ, Christ stated the obvious: "Your faith has made you well." As they accepted the invitation to believe and headed off to show the priests that their leprous bodies had been healed, the power of our living God renewed their skin and they were healed. The process still works today. A step in faith can bring healing.

Another example is when Naaman asked Elisha to cure his leprosy; he had to surrender his control and self-sufficiency. Elisha sent a messenger to Naaman, who told him to wash himself seven times in the Jordan and his flesh would be restored. Naaman was not a happy camper. He was irritated that Elisha didn't lay hands on him and cure him immediately. He didn't want to spend any more time in the land of his enemies. The miracle from God was ready to happen; all Naaman had to do was believe and get in the water seven times. He had to get past his pride and let faith take over.

Being a parent of children with ADHD, severe dyslexia, seizures, speech issues, obsessive-compulsive disorder, allergies, precocious puberty, as well as social and developmental delays brought me to my knees. Overwhelmed with all of their issues and truly with only the faith of a mustard seed, I trusted God for direction and healing. It took their entire childhood to reach the priests, but with each year, God renewed their bodies and my faith grew. I had to get past my overwhelming fatigue and my inability to solve all their problems, and allow God to use me to serve not only my kids but eventually hundreds seeking another way to health. We learned early on that Ritalin was not a good thing for our kids. As a person who loves learning, I leaped into the natural healing adventure with gusto. I gathered every book and researched every folk medicine cure available. I watched the hand of God carry my hubby and me through full-time jobs and meeting the needs of three very special, high-maintenance children. We found our quiet time each morning with God provided us the manna we needed a day at a time. My natural protocol became a common-sense approach of affirming God's power, building up the body, getting rid of the junk that causes havoc inside our bodies, and directing energy to specific weak areas.

It's not easy for kids to understand that you are what you eat. And at Halloween when everyone was gobbling down candy, we opted for a new toy or a trip to the movies instead of the sugar-collecting ritual observed by other families. Throwing out the convenient sugar-laden boxes of cereal and eating protein for breakfast every morning increased our kids' ability to concentrate at school and lessened the stress on them and me! Knowing that constipation is the number one cause for meltdowns, we were diligent about fluids and fiber. Sometimes we had use smoke and mirrors to get compliance. Everyone knows that bigger is better, so prunes became "big raisins" in our home. Each small action brought huge returns on their ability to learn at school and be healthy. It is important to note that healing looks different from God's perspective. Our kids have issues they will deal with the rest of their lives. However, they have been richly blessed, and I am so proud of them.

God's adventure led me to return to school at age fifty-seven, and I received my certification from the American Naturopathic Medical Board four years later as a Board Certified Doctor of Naturopathic Medicine. Once again, it was truly a miracle of God, since it had been decades since I had graduated from college and the gray matter really struggled through each course. It's wonderful to look back to see how God's blueprint for my life has lead me here; and now in my sixties, I know that there's much more to come.

As a classical naturopath, I believe in allopathic—traditional—medicine, and see myself as a complimentary, as opposed to an alternative, practitioner. If I'm in a car wreck, don't give me an apple; take me to the ER! I like to work with my patient's doctors to find ways to improve their health. My goal as a naturopath is to serve as the original meaning of doctor: a teacher. I want to help people understand the holistic concept of health and to expand my passion for the use of herbs as medicine.

Jesus, with open arms, brings God's welcome to every sick soul. The truth found in Jesus's ministry was that everyone is sick; no one is well. Jesus insisted that He came for those who are sick, not for those who are well. The question is whether or not we'll allow ourselves to step out in faith and be embraced by the Healer.

Introduction

> For you were bought at a price, therefore glorify God in your body and in your Spirit, which are God's.
>
> —1 Cor 6:20

In a new report, the World Health Organization estimates that the number of cancer cases will increase by 70 percent over the next two decades.[1] Currently, 14 million people worldwide are diagnosed with cancer each year, and this could reach 24 million per year by 2035. Each year in the United States, 1.6 million people are diagnosed with cancer and more than five hundred and eighty thousand will die from the disease. Breast cancer is the most frequently diagnosed cancer and the leading cause of cancer death among females, with 23 percent of total cancer cases and 14 percent of cancer deaths. Lung cancer is the leading cancer in males, with 17 percent of the total cancer cases and 23 percent of cancer deaths.

---

[1]   Sarah Bosely, "Cancer Cases expected to increase 70%", posted 2/03/14, guardian,co.uk

The Cancer Research Fund indicates there is an alarming level of naivety about diet's role in cancer. Most people believe cancer is mainly due to family history, but the World Cancer Research Fund says no more than 10 percent of cancers are due to inherited genes. According to the American Cancer Society, "Some cases of cancer are caused by an abnormal gene that is being passed along from generation to generation. Although this is often referred to as *inherited* cancer, what is inherited is the abnormal gene that can lead to cancer, not the cancer itself. Only about 5 percent to 10 percent of all cancers are inherited—resulting directly from gene defects (called mutations) inherited from a parent."[2]

When someone has inherited an abnormal copy of a gene, their cells already start out with one mutation. This makes it all the easier (and quicker) for enough mutations to build up for a cell to become cancer. That is why cancers that are inherited tend to occur earlier in life than cancers of the same type that are not inherited.

Cancer is such a common disease that it is no surprise that many families have at least a few members who have had cancer. Sometimes, certain types of cancer seem to run in some families. This can be caused by a number of factors. It can be because family members have certain risk factors in common, such as smoking, which can cause many types of cancer. It can also be due in part to some other factors, like

---

[2]   "Family Cancer Syndromes", American Cancer Society, http://cancer.org/cancer/cancercauses/geneticsandcancer

obesity, that tend to run in families and influence cancer risk.

With the cost of treatment of cancers spiraling out of control, prevention is absolutely critical, and it's been somewhat neglected. Cancer costs are projected to reach $158 billion by 2020[3]. We need to focus on cancer prevention by tackling diet and lifestyle. "People seem to mistakenly accept their chances of getting cancer as a throw of the dice, but making lifestyle changes today can help prevent cancer tomorrow," commented Chris Wild Director of WHO Research Agency on Cancer.[4] So even if you have an abnormal gene, with intentional work on your part, you have a good chance of not becoming another cancer statistic.

So the good news is you probably won't get cancer if you have a healthy lifestyle.

Prevention is basically five steps: A,B,C,D,E

- Affirmation of a higher power to activate your healing response
- Building up your body from the cellular level
- Cleaning out the waste

---

[3] National Institutes of Health, "Cancer costs projected to reach at least $158 billion in 2020". Accessed March 23, 2015. http://www.cancer.gov/newscenter/newsfromnci/.2011/costcancer

[4] Sarah Boseley, "Cancer cases expected to increase 70" over next 20 years", The Guradian

- Directly supporting your body with regular healthy activities
- Evaluate your health regularly

It is important to understand the cause of disease. Our body's health is dependent on how healthy our cells are. Cells are made up of atoms. When these atoms are healthy, the cells replicate and keep the body well and disease free. A cell must have paired electrons to be healthy. Atoms missing electrons (known as free radicals) destroy surrounding atoms by stealing their electrons. Free radicals alter or destroy cells as well as damage DNA, which creates the seed for disease. Cells that replicate in a damaged state create disease.

So the question we all want to ask is, how do you get free radicals?

Free radicals play a dual role as both beneficial and toxic compounds. The birth and death of cells in the body goes on continuously. It is a process that is necessary to keep the body healthy. Yet there is a downside. While the body metabolizes oxygen very efficiently, 1–2 percent of cells will get damaged in the process and turn into free radicals. They are produced either from this normal cell metabolism or from external sources. Endogenous or free radicals from metabolism are formed from immune cell activation, inflammation, mental stress, excessive exercise, infection, cancer, and aging. Exogenous free radicals are from external sources, such as air and water pollution, cigarette smoke, alcohol, heavy or transition metals, medications, drugs, industrial solvents, smoked meat, and radiation. In addition, we eat foods that increase oxidation and inflammation, such as refined sugar, white flour, hydrogenated oils, trans fats, and food additives. This reminds me of a fellow naturopath who said, "The whiter your bread, the sooner you're dead."

After penetration into the body, these exogenous compounds are decomposed or metabolized into free radicals. A low or moderate level can exert beneficial effects on cellular responses and immune function. They can act as weapons for our defense system. Free radicals are released by our immune system to destroy invading pathogenic microbes to fight against disease. A high concentration of free radicals generates oxidative stress, which is a process that can damage all cell structures. According to the International Journal of Biomedical Science[5], oxidative stress plays a major part in the development of chronic and degenerative ailments, such as cancer, arthritis, aging, autoimmune disorders, and cardiovascular and neurodegenerative diseases.

Cancer is the abnormal growth of cells. Humans are made up of about 75 trillion cells that continually replicate themselves. Each cell has a set of genetic instructions in its center, called *DNA*, that controls cell growth, development, and replication. When the DNA gets damaged, it can replicate an altered cell. When this altered cell replicates itself, this becomes cancer. Free radicals damage DNA. Most scientists believe it is free radical damage to the DNA

---

[5]   Lee-Young Chau, "Heme Oxygenase-1: emerging target of cancer therapy". Journal of Biomedical Science 22 (2015); doi:10.1186/s12929-015-0128-0.

that begins many forms of cancer. Two-time Nobel Prize winner for his work with cells, Dr. Otto Warburg, found that cancerous cells have lost all their genetically programmed instructions. They only know how to replicate—grow!

Antioxidants to the rescue.

Antioxidants protect DNA from damage caused by free radicals. In addition, some antioxidants can actually repair damaged DNA before it replicates. Besides protecting DNA, antioxidants also give an extra electron to the free radical. The free radical is neutralized, and the chain reaction of damage stops. Antioxidants are naturally produced in our bodies or found in whole foods, such as fruits, vegetables, nuts, oils, and beans, dietary beta-carotene and lycopene, or through supplements, such as vitamins C and E. They act as free radical scavengers by preventing and repairing damage caused by free radicals. They enhance the immune defense and lower the risk of cancer and degenerative diseases. The free radicals should equal the number of antioxidants in our body. When an antioxidant destroys a free radical, this antioxidant itself becomes destroyed. Therefore, the antioxidant resources must be constantly restored in the body. The goal is to keep a balance in life, especially when it comes to controlling free radical damage. Seems pretty simple to me: a diet of foods full of antioxidants can help prevent cancer.

A typical person consumes only one and a half servings of vegetables and no fruit each day. And as a reminder, ketchup and a piece of wilted lettuce on a hamburger does not equal a vegetable serving. Unfortunately, most people eat processed produce (canned or frozen, where the antioxidant value is lost in the processing) if they eat any at all. There really is a reason for that. The produce at the grocery store has been picked green and shipped to the store. That means it's never been allowed to develop its full flavor or antioxidant value. Seek out locally grown produce at farmer's markets, grow your own, or seek out organic produce for the best antioxidant investment for your health.

There must be two factors existing for you to develop cancer. You must have free radical damage causing a low-oxygen environment that encourages the development of anaerobic cells, and your immune system must be weakened so that it is not able to recognize and destroy these cells. Through some basic changes in your life, you can empower your immune system to function at its best and limit free radical damage to your cells.

Cancer has been accepted as an unfortunate but inevitable fact of life. *So not true.* Diseases are not caught but caused by what we eat or don't eat. We are masters of our destiny. We control the health of our cells through what we eat. Yes, you are truly what you eat!

Step 1

Affirming Faith to Activate Healing in Our Bodies

Faith Activates Healing

> Trust in the Lord with all your heart, and
> lean not on your own understanding.
>
> —Proverbs 3:5

The very word *cancer* brings great fear—fear and helplessness.
God understands our fear. Before we were born, His Holy
Spirit inspired men to give us a tool to help counter fear.
He has written 115 times in the Bible, "Do not fear," or
"Fear not." Having a stronger faith will empower you to
trust more and fear less. We are works in progress. We
won't be completely free of fear until we reach heaven.
Meanwhile, each day we must choose to lay everything
in God's hands. God tells us that He knows the number
of hairs on our heads and the number of days in our lives
(Psalm 139:13–16). Our fear will not change the length of
our lives, only the quality. We need to let go of all the things
that seem urgent and more important—e-mails, television
programs, texting, social media, phone calls—and make
regular contact with God.

David Servan-Schreiber, MD, PhD, shares in his book *Anti-Cancer, A New Way of Life,*[6] that this emotion of fear and helplessness actually causes the body to respond in a negative way that causes inflammation in the body. Researchers in the new field of psychoneuroimmunology have found that feelings of helplessness cause the release of hormones that activate the body's inflammatory response, which can facilitate the growth and spread of tumors. Additionally, stress slows down the functions of digestion, tissue repair, and immunity.

We all have cancer in our bodies. One definition of cancer is the breakdown in the balance between cancer cells that have always been dormant in the body and the natural defenses that normally keep them at bay. Dr. Servan-Schreiber calls cancer cells "armed bandits, roving outside the law." One way to keep them dormant is stop the inflammation that they need to grow. A solid relationship with the Creator of the universe can help stop these bandits before they multiply and invade neighboring cells.

More faith also brings dependence on God, so helplessness can actually be a good thing. Our Creator knows we cannot handle the cluster bomb of chaos that radiates into our lives. We were designed to be helpless. We cannot live without the protection God provides to buffer the damage from the world around us. Believing that God is truly in control is a way of redistributing stress off our shoulders and onto His.

---

[6]   David Servan-Schreiber MD, PhD, Anti Cancer: A New Way of Life. New York: Penguin Group Inc. 2009

Several studies with mice have clearly indicated that feelings of helplessness feed cancer. The study by Martin Seligman, PhD, at the University of Pennsylvania in 1982 found that it isn't the stress itself that promotes cancer development but the persistent perception of helplessness we may have in the face of stress that affects the body's reaction to the disease. The opposite has also been shown to be true. A state of serenity will slow down cancerous growth.

Each sunrise brings us the opportunity to trust God more and improve our health. Trust is not comprehensive. It is an intentional commitment we must make each day. It is an act of the mind and the body. To shore up our faith against the waves of anxiety and stress hitting us every day, we must think, *I trust God, and I have no fear,* and we must also say it whenever the waves reach us. Scientific studies by Dr. Luciano Bernardi[7] at the University of Pavia, Italy, have examined the automatic body rhythms of heart rate, blood pressure, respiration, etc., and found that when balanced, they promote good health. Dr. Bernardi tested a control group by asking them to repeat a text they knew by heart, thus requiring no mental effort or stress. He found that when they repeated the rosary at a frequency of six breaths per minute, all the different biological rhythms being measured became mutually balanced. Researchers at Ohio State University and the National institutes of Health published a study reviewing all the studies regarding the amplitude and variations of biological rhythms. They

---

[7]   L P Bernaardi, MD, "Effect of Rosary Prayer and Yoga Mantras on autonomic Cardiovascular Rhythms". British Medical Journal 343 (2001):1446-49.

found three specific health benefits: better functioning of the immune system, reduction of inflammation, and better regulation of blood sugar levels.

So just by saying, "I trust God, and I have no fear," or your favorite Bible verse six times, exhaling as you say it, you can reset your breathing, allowing more oxygen into your body, and bring all your body systems out of alert and back to normal. This will prevent free radical damage and stop cancer from growing in your body. Preventing the destruction of your body at the cellular level each and every day is the best way to prevent cancer. Nutrition and making good lifestyle choices definitely help, but only when you live your life with the joyful peace that comes from completely trusting God will you have vibrant health.

Positive Thinking

> A merry heart does good, like medicine, but
> a broken spirit dries the bones.
>
> —Proverbs 17:22

It's a fact. If you wake up in the morning and think you're going to have a bad day, you will have a bad day. Negative thinkers tend to begin a day thinking something will go wrong. Instead, focus on the aspects of your day that could go right and what you are looking forward to about your day. Negative attitudes come from negative thoughts, which come from reactions to negative behavior. Few will argue with the fact that people simply are happier and feel more optimistic when they have positive thoughts. Thoughts and emotions are vibrations or energies, which have a ripple effect that runs through the whole body, creating a response—positive or negative.

Bad things happen. When they do, positive thinkers look at the situation realistically, search for ways they can improve the situation, and try to learn from their experiences. You have a choice. You can focus on a thought that makes you feel bad or focus on a thought that makes you feel good. Focus your energy on positive thinking and ways to make your life more enjoyable, and you may discover that positive thinking really does help you feel better.

Choose to be optimistic and enjoy the many health benefits of optimism. Positive thinking helps a person to enjoy life by having a healthy outlook and attitude when life's adversities come along. Your outlook on life helps to reduce your stress level, boost your self-esteem, and even improve your health, according to the Mayo Clinic[8]. Additional health benefits include lesser rates of depression, improved resistance to the common cold, and reduced risk of cardiovascular disease. An ongoing study of one hundred thousand women funded by the National Institutes of Health[9] found that negative-thinking women were 23 percent more likely to die from cancer.

Steps to Positive Thinking

Make a list of things you are grateful for: Gratitude is an amazing emotion in that it is almost impossible to feel negative thoughts when you are focusing on things you are grateful for. Motivational speaker Tony Robbins says that no

[8] "Positive thinking: stop negative self-talk to reduce stress", Mayo Clinic, accessed March 23, 2015, http://www.mayoclinic.org/healthy-living/stress-management.

[9] Jerry Shaw, "Health Benefits of Positive Thinking", Livestrong.com, accessed Jan.28, 2015, http://www.livestrong.com/article/75627-health-benefits-positive-thinking/.

matter how much money you have, if you are not grateful, you are poor. Thank God each day for five things.

Exercise: The Mayo Clinic reports that exercising at least three times a week can produce a positive mood. Walking is the best exercise to boost your spirits. Breathe deeply and smile while you're walking.

Find positive friends: Surrounding yourself with positive people will help you find the encouragement you need to live a positive life. Everyone knows someone who is refreshingly fun to be around. These people seem to naturally maintain a positive attitude, and negative, faithless words do not cross their lips. They are beacons, and many are drawn to them. So stop hanging around with people who do nothing but spout negative stuff.

Cut back on the nightly news: So much negative news is reported by the media. Expose yourself to an abundance of negativity, and you will begin to be more negative. Limit yourself to the first five minutes of headlines and move on.

Pray for the power that passes all understanding: You can't change the habit of negative thinking by yourself. Remember to spend time with the one who is able to help. Do what you can, and let God do the rest.

Rest and Relaxation

> Thus the heavens and the earth, and all the host of them, were finished. And on the seventh day God ended His work, which He had done, and He rested on the seventh day from all His work which He had done. Then God blessed the seventh day and sanctified it, because in it He rested from all His work, which God had created and made.
>
> —Genesis 2:1–3

Rest is repeated throughout Scripture, beginning with creation. God created the earth in six days, and then He rested. He rested not because He was tired but to set a standard for humankind to follow. The Ten Commandments made resting on the Sabbath a requirement (Exodus 20:8–11). God is serious about rest. To rest, we have to trust God to take care of things for us. Since one definition of *relax* is "to become less firm," then giving our lives, careers, and families to God is the best way to relax. Rest and relaxation are gifts from God, given so we might grow closer to Him.

Rest simply means to cease work or activity. In our fast-paced world, many of us have lost the importance of rest. It is one of the most vital needs we have. Every day, the body moves and performs bodily processes. Without rest, the muscles and all the other parts of the body will eventually wear out. Rest allows the body to restore energy that has been expended from our day-to-day work. It revitalizes all the systems in the body to maintain the body's optimum level of functioning.

"It is important to engage in multiple leisure activities, both as a way to enjoy life more, but also to potentially have a benefit on health and be a stress reliever," reported Karen Matthews of the University of Pittsburgh's Mind-Body Center[10]. "People who had more leisure activities reported more life satisfaction, finding more meaning in life," says Matthews. "They tended to be more religious and spiritual in orientation. They reported having a lot of support from friends as well as having a large network of friends and family."

Another great source for relaxation is laughter. Feeling rundown? Try laughing more. Many medical professionals think laughter just might be the best medicine, helping you feel better and putting that spring back in your step. Laughter helps you relax and recharge. It reduces stress and increases energy, enabling you to stay focused and accomplish more. Our body changes physiologically when

---

[10]   Jerry Shaw, "Health Benefits of Positive Thinking", Livestrong. com, last up0dated Jan 28, 2015, http://livestrong.com/ article/75627-health-benefits-positive-thinking/.

we laugh. We stretch muscles throughout our face and body, our pulse and blood pressure go up, and we breathe faster, sending more oxygen to our tissues. Researchers at the University of Maryland[11] have shown that the ability to use humor may raise the level of infection-fighting antibodies in the body, thus improving your resistance to disease.

Use every opportunity to laugh:

Watch a funny movie or TV show; read the funny pages; share a joke or funny story; play with a pet; play with a child and make time for fun activities, such as bowling, miniature golf, game night etc. These things will help your health. And don't forget to smile! It is the beginning of laughter, and it is contagious.

Most people do not get enough sleep, and the rest they do get is not full and deep sleep. According to the Harvard Women's Health Watch[12], more people are sleeping less than six hours per night, and sleep difficulties visit 75 percent of us at least a few nights a week. Without proper rest, we cannot recharge our cells. Tired cells cannot eliminate toxins efficiently. It is during rest that most healing takes place. The pattern of waking up, working all day non-stop, going to bed late, and never getting a full, deep eight hours of peaceful sleep results in a body that slowly begins to break

---

[11]   "Give Your Body a Boost – With Laughter", WebMD, accessed Mar 23, 2015. http://www.webmd.com/balance/features/give-your-body-boost.

[12]   "Importance of sleep: Six reasons not to scrimp on sleep", Harvard Health Publications, last modified Jan 1,2006, hhtp://www.health.harvard.edu/press_releases/imporantce of sleep.

down and never has a chance to heal and recharge. The body is much like a battery utilizing electric current. It must be given a chance to rest and recharge to work properly. If a person did nothing else but get proper sleep, their energy levels would skyrocket and the amount of illness and disease they experienced would go down. Sleep deprivation alters immune function, including the activity of the body's killer cells. Keeping up with sleep may also help fight cancer.

Most of us know that eight hours of sleep per night is optimal. But what many people don't realize is that the actual time you fall asleep is important too. The best rest is when the sun is no longer shining. Sleeping from one a.m. to nine a.m. is not as restorative as sleeping from ten p.m. to six a.m. The reason why is because hormone secretion, body temperature, digestion, and other important restorative processes follow a twenty-four-hour cycle linked to natural light exposure. The later in the evening we fall asleep and the later in the morning we wake up, the more out-of-sync our cycle becomes.

Most people toss and turn at night. The ideal situation is that you virtually do not move for the entire sleep time. When sleep is full and deep, brainwave activity can occur, which stimulates the healing process throughout the body.

To promote good sleep, add foods containing tryptophan, which promotes sleep, to your evening meal: bananas, dates, figs, milk, nut butters, tuna, turkey, wholegrain crackers, or yogurt.

Stress Management

> Though the fig tree may not blossom, Nor fruit be on the vines; Though the labor of the olive may fail, And the fields yield no food; Though the flock may be cut off from the fold, And there be no herd in the stalls—Yet I will rejoice in the Lord, I will joy in the God of my salvation.
>
> —Habakkuk 3:17-19

Today there is a tsunami of reasons for worry, tension, anxiety, and stress. We all face issues, from unpaid bills to family arguments, that help build stress in our bodies. The Institute of Science, Technology & Public Policy[13] reports that leading medical experts estimate that 90 percent of disease is caused or complicated by stress.

Our feelings of stress or anxiety may be our mind's way of telling us to attend to our spiritual needs. Ecclesiastes assures

---

[13] The Congressional Prevention Coalition, "Stress Prevention". Institute of Science, Technology and Public Policy, Presented June 24, 1998, http://istpp.org/coalition/stress_prevention.html

us that there is a time for everything—work and rest. We are limited by time and energy. We really can't do everything, and we weren't made to do everything. So cease striving. Our problems are usually perceptual. Our problems seem really big, because our God seems really small. Our biggest problem really is that we have an inadequate understanding of who God is. The first step to managing our stress is to increase the size of our God.

Tozer said[14], "A low view of God … is the cause of a hundred lesser evils. However if you view God as able to do anything and really believe it, you are relieved of ten thousand temporal problems."

God tells us in Isaiah 55:9 that "as the heavens are higher than the earth, so are my thoughts higher than your thoughts." I have a hard time wrapping my mind around the thought of celestial beings light years away. Astronomers have spied galaxies 12.3 billion light years form earth. To better understand, the light from the sun is only eight minutes old, but the light from the farthest galaxy that we know about takes 12.3 billion years to get here. God is so much bigger than we can even imagine. Refocusing our minds on the bigness of God makes our problems small.

With God, there is no middle ground; either you believe He is able or you don't. When you finally focus on His magnificent power, not only with your heart but with your

---

[14] A.W. Tozer, "Created To Worship God", WordPress.com, updated Dec 1, 2011, https://psalm86nine.wordpress.com/2011/12/01.quote-from-tozer/

mind, you release the power of the stress in your life. To release the stress, you have to not only think it, but you have to say it. Verbalizing, "God, your power and greatness is more than I can understand, and I know you have my life in your hands. All knowing God, you have everything under your control." I think Zechariah 4:6 says it best: "Not by might nor by power, but by my Spirit says the Lord Almighty."

Much stress is related to our feeling of helplessness or lack of control. Christians can take great comfort in knowing that God remains in control of our lives, using even stress for good to develop our stamina and character. Rather than allowing situations to control us, we can by God's power rise above the situation and turn it around for our own good (Rom 5:3-6).

What happens when our God is too small?
Our adrenal glands send out first responders.

When the brain perceives stress, it sends a chemical message to the pituitary, which releases a hormone, which causes the adrenals to start producing epinephrine (adrenaline) and cortisol. Epinephrine, a hormone and neurotransmitter, causes the fight-or-flight response. It tenses our muscles, increases our heart rate and blood pressure, dilates the bronchial, speeds up our breathing, and shuts down digestion and anything else not essential for survival. Cortisol is good for your body in moderation. It reduces inflammation, helping your body to deal with injury and pain. When too much is released in your body, it depresses the immune function (critical for preventing cancer), raises blood sugar levels, and doesn't allow the body to relax and sleep at night. The major cause of night terrors in both adults and children is too much cortisol in the blood at bedtime. Obviously, long-term stress has a huge impact on our health. Major issues include poor digestion, constipation, tension headaches, neck and shoulder pain, low back pain, ulcers, high blood pressure, blood clotting, increased risk of infections, asthma, diabetes, excess weight, as well as cancer. Good health requires destressing yourself.

Tips

* Fun

When I recommend an hour of relaxation every week for my patients, the reaction is always surprising. Most say they don't have time, but they clearly like the idea. Often, busy mothers break down in tears and say they really could use an hour to themselves. Only when I say it is "doctor's orders" do they smile and say they will try to make it happen. If you continue to wear down, it not only hurts you but it hurts your family, your employer—everyone suffers.

* Breathe Deeply

When stressed, we tend to hold our breath or shallow breathe. Quick, short, inhales of air do not provide the oxygen our body requires. Intentional, deep inhales will bring much-needed oxygen and will cause our muscles to relax. Try the 1-2-3 breathing method when stressed. Breathe in while counting 1-2-3, hold 1-2-3, and exhale 1-2-3 until you feel calm.

• Exercise

The stress hormones get us ready to run away or activate the caveman response of physically fighting our way out of our problem. In other words we are geared up for physical exercise. Often our sedentary lifestyles do not give our bodies an outlet for all this pent-up energy. Only through regular exercise can we de-stress our bodies.

• Aid with Adaptagens

Adaptogens are herbs that have been found to greatly reduce the impact of stress on our health. Adaptagenic herbs modulate the signals that are sent from the hypothalamus and pituitary glands, causing a reduction of adrenal output of adrenaline and cortisol, thus lowering overall stress levels. They help to break damaging fight-or-flight chain reaction patterns caused by stress. Herbs that have been identified as possessing adaptogenic properties include American and Korean ginseng, eleuthro root (Siberian ginseng), maca and suma.

• Other supplements

Getting control of your nerves requires good fats, such as butter, coconut oil, nuts, olive oil, flax seed oil, and Omega-3 essential fatty acids. Consider adding a B complex to your diet to help you cope with stress.

"Do not fear" or "Fear not" are used 115 times in the Bible. Listen to God and live abundantly! Be still before God and let His Light permeate your thinking. Nurture your body, mind, and soul by communing with God regularly.

Step 2

Building the Body

Building the Body Overview

> Do not be deceived. A man reaps what he
> sows.
>
> Gal 6:7

Our lives are constantly besieged by busyness, hurry, and
noise. Living full-throttle is expected, while running on
empty is the norm. The majority of people I see in my
practice are tired and stressed. The number one goal, hands
down, when I work with a patient to create a health plan is
more energy.

Every day, people come into my office asking, "Why do I
always feel so exhausted?" Once we review their lifestyle
and fueling options for their body, it is clear why they are
running on low. When it comes to health, we reap what
we sow. Each of us need to learn to make choices that give
the protective and healing powers in our bodies a fighting
chance.

Our bodies are self-repairing mechanisms. The nature of
our makeup, starting at the cellular level, has been created

for self-repair. Approximately 97 percent of the cells in our body are replaced every year from the food we eat. Food is the energy needed for healing. Healing is constantly taking place in the human body. Antioxidants in our body rescue damaged cells; white blood cells rush to capture and cut off viral and bacterial invaders; the liver is constantly removing excess hormones or fat from our system; our skin forms a scab when we cut our finger. We are a healing machine! All of this happens because of the body's God-given ability to heal itself. God expects us to care for the physical bodies and not neglect or abuse them in any way. If we don't take care of our bodies and this causes disease, such as cancer, then we must be willing to change our lifestyle, with God's help.

The immune system is not a single organ but the whole body working together. It is like building your house on a firm rock where life's storms cannot shake you. As a Christian and as a doctor of naturopathic medicine, I am concerned about the incidence of cancer exploding in our country. Statistics clearly show that one out of every three people will develop some form of cancer in his or her lifetime. That's a third of our population—a tsunami of cancer heading our way. Every year, hundreds of billions of dollars are spent on cancer treatment and research. Yet the numbers continue to grow. Now is the time to focus on prevention.

We all want to live healthy and disease-free forever. Truly healthy people are full of energy and vitality. The good news is that when all your systems are running at optimal levels you can have vibrant dynamic health.

Here's a basic tip to build your body to its peak capacity: eat more fresh, organic fruits and veggies. The biggest change you can make in your life is to eat five servings of veggies and two pieces of fruit every day! Consider buying a juicer and drink a glass of raw, uncooked, awesome power full of enzymes, vitamins and minerals, nutrition, and life force.

Antioxidants

> Then they shall eat the flesh on that night,
> roasted in the fire with unleavened bread
> and with bitter herbs they shall eat it.
>
> —Exodus 12:38

Long before scientists could break down a plant into its molecular components, God provided mankind with information about foods He wanted us to eat.

Antioxidants are nature's way of fighting off potentially dangerous molecules in the body. Antioxidants' sole purpose are to neutralize free radicals. The primary food source of all antioxidants is plant foods. Fruits and vegetables provide the body with antioxidants needed to properly wage war against free radicals.

The best way to get a variety of antioxidants in the diet is to eat foods that represent all the colors of the rainbow. Each color provides its own unique antioxidant effects.

Bright orange and deep yellow fruits and vegetables, like carrots, sweet potatoes, and apricots, provide one type of antioxidant. Red foods, like tomatoes, provide another. Green vegetables, such as broccoli and cabbage, and blue or purple foods, like blueberries and eggplant, each have their own antioxidant packages.

USDA scientists analyzed antioxidant levels in more than one hundred different foods. Each food was measured for antioxidant concentration as well as antioxidant capacity per serving size. Cranberries, blueberries, and blackberries ranked highest among the fruits studied. Beans, artichokes, and Russet potatoes were tops among the vegetables. Pecans, walnuts, and hazelnuts ranked highest in the nut category. It is important to note that total antioxidant capacity does not necessarily reflect their health benefit. Benefits depend on how the food's antioxidants are absorbed and utilized in the body.

The following are examples of five powerful antioxidants:

- Carotenoids neutralize free radicals and enhance immune system—food sources: deeply pigmented fruits and vegetables, like carrots, dark leafy greens, sweet potatoes, kale, spinach, tomatoes, turnip and mustard greens.
- Flavonoids contribute to maintenance of brain functions; contribute to heart health; strengthen antioxidant cell defenses; and increase immune defenses—food sources: apples, apricots, blueberries, citrus fruits, pears, plumes, raspberries, strawberries, beans, cabbage, onions, green tea, purple grapes.

- Isothiocyanates enhance detoxification and deactivate carcinogens—food sources: cruciferous vegetables, like cabbage, broccoli, cauliflower, kale, turnips, collards, Brussels sprouts, Bok Choy, radishes, kohlrabi, watercress.
- Resveratrol protect the lining of blood vessels in the heart and reduce inflammation—food sources: dark chocolate, mulberries, red wine, red and purple grapes and juice, peanuts, blueberries, cranberries.
- Tannins have potent antiviral, antibacterial, and anti-parasitic effects—food sources: cocao powder, pomegranates, chickpeas, cashews, walnuts, lentils, green tea, barley.

Fruits and vegetables containing phytochemicals have been found to inhibit cancer growth. Phytochemical compounds are molecules produced by plants that repair the damage caused by aggressors and allow the plant to survive. Studies have shown they interfere with the sequence of events that cause tumor growth. They are antioxidants on steroids.

Consider consumption of one of these foods each day for cancer prevention:

blueberries	green tea
broccoli	soybeans
cabbage	strawberries
citrus	tomatoes
garlic	turmeric
grapes	

We know that 30 percent of all cancers are from poor dietary habits. And according to the World Health Organization[15], cancer is not evenly distributed throughout the world. The countries with the highest incidence of cancer are those in Eastern Europe, with 300-400 cases per 100,000 inhabitants, closely followed by the Western industrialized nations of the United States and Canada, with 260 cases per 100,000 inhabitants.

Eating your fruits and vegetables may not prevent cancer or many other diseases, but it can give your body the fighting chance that it needs. The benefits of getting your daily dose of fruits and vegetables are numerous! Keep in mind, the fresher your produce, the more antioxidants.

---

[15]   Sarah Bosely, "Cancer cases expected to increase 70% over next 20 years", The Guardian, posted Feb 03, 2014, http://www.theguardian.com/society/2014/feb/03/worldwide-cancer-cases-soar-next-20-years.

Essential Fatty Acids

> You eat the fat, wear the wool and butcher
> the fattened animals, but you do not tend
> the flock.
>
> —Ezekiel 34:3

Despite all the propaganda against fats, we need them in our diet to stay healthy. Fats play a critical role in our health. Brain and nerve tissue require the proper kind of fats, and low-fat diets impact our ability to properly use our brains. The heart burns fat as its primary source of fuel. Fats are burned to keep the body warm in cold weather and are necessary for the production of many hormones. Extremely low-fat diets are not good for us and may actually raise cholesterol levels, because about half of the cholesterol in our bodies is needed to make bile to digest fats.

Essential fatty acids are considered essential because the human body cannot synthesize them. They are only derived from food. Two kinds of essential fatty acids are omega-3s and omega-6s. Both are needed in our bodies but should be properly balanced to promote good health and build the immune system. They help form cells walls, aid the heart, and fight depression. If they are not in proper balance, you can experience blood clots, memory issues, irregular heartbeat, and a weak immune system. The differing numbers identifying omega-3 and omega-6 fatty acids simply refer to where the carbon-carbon double bonds are positioned in the molecules. The recommended ratio is one omega-3 fat to four omega-6 fats. Omega -3 fatty acids help reduce inflammation, and most omega-6 fatty acids tend to promote inflammation. An inappropriate balance of these essential fatty acids contributes to the development of disease while a proper balance helps maintain and even improve health.

With the Western diet of over-processed foods, we end up with too many omega-6 fats and not enough omega-3 fats (estimated daily consumption is 1:25 which is way past the recommended 1:4 ratio). The abundance of omega-6 fatty acids over omega-3 explains the rising rate of inflammatory disorders, such as cancer, in the United States. Because both fatty acids compete for each other to be converted to active metabolites (pro-inflammatory and anti-inflammatory) in the body, decreasing the intake of omega-6 fatty acids and increasing dietary omega-3 fatty acids is generally considered beneficial. Omega-6 fatty acids are known to trigger the onset of cancer, but including omega-3s in the diet of lab rats slowed down the development of breast, colon, prostate, and pancreatic cancers.

Omega-3 fatty acids can be found in fat fish, like wild salmon, tuna, halibut, sardines and Pollock, also in krill, algae, walnut, nut oils, coconut, olive oil, avocado, and flaxseed.

Build Your Body with Good Food

> Their fruits will be used for food and their
> leaves for medicine.
>
> —Ezekiel 47:12

So many of us live under the false belief that cancer is just a game of luck. Getting cancer is not just the roll of the dice. Our way of life creates an environment for mutated and possibly cancerous cells to grow.

Every day, we are making choices that will either protect us from getting cancer or will make us more susceptible to the disease. Our eating habits are one of the major factors in cancer growth or cancer starvation and elimination. Three to five times each day, we eat meals. That is three to five times a day that we mentally decide what we are putting in our bodies. The problem comes when what our bodies need and what our taste buds want don't exactly align.

Current Western surveys of nutrition show that 56 percent of our calories come from three sources: refined sugars (cane and beet sugar, corn syrup, etc.), bleached flour (white bread, white pasta, etc.), and vegetable oils (soybean, sunflower, corn, and trans-fats). None of these three sources contain any of the proteins, vitamins, minerals, and omega-3 fatty acids that our bodies require to function, but the one thing that they do nurture is cancerous cells.

Researchers found a significant difference in cancer rates in the West compared to Eastern nations. According to the World Cancer Research Cancer Foundation, the United States is ranked in the top ten for the highest rate of cancer in both men and women, securely holding down the number six spot. Japan barely made it into the top fifty, at the forty-eighth position, and China was not even in the top fifty countries, having one of the lowest cancer rates in the world.

One of the major differences between these two groups of people is their beverage consumption. In the East, the second most consumed beverage following water is green tea. Green tea is a powerful antioxidant. For over twenty years, soda pop has been the number one drink in the United States, with per capita consumption peaking at fifty-four gallons a year in 1998 according to Beverage Digest.[16] Finally in 2013, increased water consumption moved America's beloved soda to second place. Filled with corn syrup, chemicals, and carbonation, soda pop not only helps promote free radical damage but provides the fuel to grow the free radical cells into long chains of cancer throughout the body.

---

[16] "Soda Studies", Beverage Digest, accessed Mar 23, 2015, http://www.beveragelife.ru/beverage-industry-statistics/sodas-studies/.

Food is both your body's fuel and the source of raw materials to produce healthy cells. Eating cheap junk food is no way to save money. It will reduce your energy and weaken your cells, and you will wind up spending far more in doctor and hospital bills than you saved by eating low quality food. Put your money into whole, natural, organically grown foods instead.

The best thing you can do to prevent cancer is to make it a habit to eat seven half-cup servings of fresh fruits and vegetables every day. It's also important to select natural sugars, such as raw honey, xylitol, organic natural brown sugar, or stevia. Many studies have shown that an overconsumption of refined sugar increases the insulin levels in our system and thereby contributes to cancer cell growth. It is therefore important to avoid foods with a high glycemic index and choose those with a low glycemic index. Note, if you find yourself craving sugar foods, you need to eat more healthy fats and proteins. Healthy fats include olive oil, organic butter and cream from grass-fed cows, coconut oil, avocados, and nuts. Not only can starting your day with a tablespoon of coconut oil reduce your sugar cravings, but it will stop acid reflux from happening.

In addition to eating whole foods, you may need to supplement with digestive enzymes to help you break down the food so you can absorb it. As we get older, we may not have enough hydrochloric acid in our stomach to properly break down the food. If you are bloating and feel gassy on a regular basis, you could have undigested food in your intestinal tract that is putrefying and causing a build up of waste and toxins. This fermentative process releases lactic acid that inhibits transportation of oxygen to neighboring cells. Make sure you find a digestive enzyme with protease, amylase, lipase, and lactase to break down proteins, fats, carbs, and dairy.

In general,

- eat grass-fed organic animal products;
- balance your diet;
- reduce your intake of sugar, white flour, products containing omega-6 essential fatty acids (sunflower oil, corn oil, soybean oil, safflower roil, margarines, hydrogenated fats);
- increase your omega-3 essential fatty acids intake (fish, grass-fed animals); and
- increase your intake of anticancer foods, like herbs, green tea, fruits, and vegetables.

Hydrate

> I am going to stand there in front of you on
> the rock of Horeb: when you hit the rock,
> water will come out of it and the people
> will drink.

> —Exodus 17:6

Hydration is essential for good health. You can live for months without food, but two to three days without water could kill you. It is estimated that 75 percent of all Americans are chronically dehydrated. On the average, water makes up 60-70 percent of your body weight. Dehydration is usually expressed as the loss of a certain percentage of one's weight. Scientists define dehydration as fluid losses greater than only 1 percent of body weight. Dehydration can become fatal when 9-12 percent of your body weight is lost via water. Our bodies are constantly losing water.

You lose water each day when you go to the bathroom, sweat, and breathe. You lose about a quart and a half of water per day just through breathing, and overall, you lose over three quarts per day. You lose water faster when the weather is really hot, when you exercise, or if you have a fever.

Signs of dehydration:

- little or no urine, or dark-colored urine
- dry mouth
- sleepiness or fatigue
- extreme thirst
- headache
- confusion
- feeling dizzy or lightheaded
- no tears when crying

It is important to note that our thirst mechanism has a lag time. Once we are thirsty, our bodies have already reached the point of moderate dehydration, and it becomes more difficult to replenish the fluids to the point of hydration.

There are different recommendations for water intake each day, but a rule of thumb is six to eight eight-ounce glasses of water each day. Water needs are also related to how many calories you burn daily. You need about 1 ml of water for every calorie you burn. So if you're very active and burn three to four thousand calories per day, you would need three to four liters of water or thirteen to seventeen cups of water. Your entire fluid intake doesn't have to come from water—fruits and veggies contain fluid and non-caffeinated beverages also can contribute to the overall total.

Tips for staying hydrated:

- Keep a bottle of water with you during the day.
- If plain water doesn't interest you, try adding a slice of lemon or lime to your drink.
- When exercising, make sure you drink water before, during, and after your workout.
- Start and end your day with a glass of water.
- When you're feeling hungry, drink water; the sensation of thirst is often confused with hunger.

Dehydration contributes to a wide variety of ailments, including indigestion, colitis, appendicitis, heartburn, rheumatoid arthritis, back and neck pain, headaches, stress, depression, high blood pressure, asthma, fatigue, memory loss, and allergies. It is a huge factor in inflammation, which is caused by free radical damage. Research indicates that eight to ten glasses of water a day could significantly ease back and joint pain for up to 80 percent of sufferers. Lack of water is the number one trigger of daytime fatigue.

Immune System

> Or do you not know that your body is the
> temple of the Holy Spirit who is in you,
> whom you have from God and you are not
> your own?
>
> —I Cor 6:19

The body normally and regularly produces cancer cells due to free radical damage. A healthy immune system recognizes and destroys these defective cells. When the immune system is unable to recognize these deviant cells or is too weak to destroy them, cancer can develop.

In today's mass-market, over-processed, and polluted world, the body needs a stronger immune system than ever before. The major factor for a weak immune system is poor nutrition. Other causes are the loss or destruction of friendly bacteria in the intestinal tract and excessive sugar consumption. Simply increasing your intake of fruits and vegetables to at least seven servings a day, decreasing your sugar intake, and adding food with probiotics will greatly improve your immune system.

Besides building immunity through input of antioxidants, large quantities of fruits and vegetables also help to alkalize the body. In order to have optimal health, the body must maintain a proper internal pH level. Cancer cells prefer an acid or anaerobic environment. Working to achieve a neutral pH of 7.0 is a great way to improve your immune system. Check body pH once a week. Use a piece of pH paper and test your saliva. If you see that your body is in the alkaline area, the chance of getting cancer or other diseases is practically zero. If you are too acidic, it's time to make some changes to get your body back into balance. Anything below 7.0 is acidic and anything above 7.0 is alkaline. The best way to create an alkaline body is to eat more vegetables!

The time is now to help the future health of the children in your family. Bolstering your child's immune system may help them have fewer sick days from school and it can also protect them from serious diseases, such as cancer, going forward.

If the immune system is strong and your children are exposed to disease, the immune system will fight off the illness and keep your child healthy. Building the body up is the major way to prevent sickness in the first place. Learning to make your lifestyle healthier and using herbs for prevention will strengthen the immune system.

In addition to increased fruits and veggies in their diets, herbs may help children to become more resistant to disease, recover faster, and make their symptoms less severe. The key to using herbs with children is finding an acceptable preparation they will take. Most children can't swallow capsules so they need a liquid dosage form.

Black elderberries (sambucus nigra) are antiviral and actually help to inhibit viruses from entering the cells. Thus they inhibit the spread of viral infections and, as an added benefit, they taste great. Just like Mary Poppins said, a teaspoon of sweetness makes the medicine go down! They are particularly good for the respiratory system. Brew berries and/or flowers as a tea and drink hot or cold daily as a prevention tool or use half to two teaspoons of a liquid extract or syrup daily. It may also be found as gummies.

One of the best herbs for the immune system is Echinacea agustifolia. It contains a substance that inhibits the spread of bacterial infection. It appears to activate and stimulate the production of white blood cells. It is the most popular herbal supplement in the United States today. You can get a liquid root extract and put one teaspoon in with another herbal syrup, like elderberry, to hide the taste. It is suggested to take one week a month to build up immunity.

Thyme is believed to stimulate the thymus gland, which regulates the immune system. It is also a powerful antiseptic and disinfectant and has been used to break up mucus and fight colds, coughs, fevers, headaches, and sore throats. The herb's name comes from *thymus*, a Greek word meaning "courage." However, you don't need to be courageous to try some thyme in the kitchen. Its aroma and taste are culinary staples of meats, salads, sauces, and soups. Use a teaspoon of thyme leaves when cooking and beef up your kid's immune system.

A whiff of catnip will remind you of mint and lemon and will make your child cat-friendly! Like many members of the mint family, it contains considerable quantities of vitamins C and E, both excellent antioxidants that fight free-radical damage, which leads to illness. It also settles the stomach and soothes the nerves. It has long been used as a remedy for colic, gas, and indigestion in children. Try a teaspoon of catnip tincture daily or brew the fresh/dried herb in hot water and drink as hot or cold tea.

Additional Key herbs to help build adult immune systems:

- Burdock—A blood-purifying herb included in many anticancer remedies. It helps the liver and lymphatics clean up morbid matter in the system.
- Chamomile—It helps settle the nerves, relieve digestive upset, and reduce inflammation. It also has anti-inflammatory action.
- Green Tea—The most commonly drunk beverage in the world next to water. It contains antioxidant compounds that prevent free-radical damage.
- Suma—Discovered in the Brazilian rain forest, it is both an adaptagen able to help the body deal with stress and an immune stimulant.
- Grape Seed—Its extract is a good source of the powerful antioxidant anthocyanin. It is effective in eliminating free radical damage.

Step 3

Cleansing

Cleansing

Every day our bodies create waste in the process of metabolism. Additionally, we put potentially harmful substances into our systems simply by eating, breathing, and drinking. In natural health, we believe our bodies are healthier if we dump the waste on a regular basis. Americans are almost fanatical about keeping the outside of our bodies clean but totally neglect cleaning the inside. Cleaning the inside is the process of getting rid of what is no longer useful and involves supporting the body's natural detoxification systems. To prevent disease, especially cancer, you absolutely must get toxins out of your body.

The best way to cleanse our body and promote spiritual growth is fasting. Fasting is a win-win. Fasting is an effective and safe method of helping the body detoxify itself and move through the releasing of toxins from the tissues into the bloodstream with greater speed and fewer symptoms. By not eating for a period of time, you relieve the body of the work of digesting foods, allowing your system to rid itself of toxins while facilitating healing. Our bodies know how to heal themselves. There is a natural process of toxin excretion, which automatically continues in our body; however, fasting accelerates the process.

Health Benefits of Fasting

- Allows the digestive system to rest—as much as 65 percent of the body's energy is needed to digest food
- Promotes cleansing and detoxification of the body
- Aids mental clarity
- Enhances spiritual connection

  And don't forget the powerful effects of fasting on our spiritual life. It forces our attention inward and gives us an opportunity to focus on the greatness of God in our lives. It is a spiritual discipline that offers the short-term effects of better health and long-term effects of spiritual growth. Combining a nutritional fast with a spiritual fast means you abstain from your regular diet while focusing on prayer.

Spiritual Benefits of Fasting

Fasting requires self-control and discipline. During fasting your focus is removed from this world and shifted to concentrate on God's power and goodness. It clears the mind and body of earthly attentions and draws us close to God. Fasting demonstrates our need for God's help and guidance through complete dependence on Him. The following Bible verses helps us to better understand reasons to fast.

- 1 Cor 9:27   It helps us connect to the Holy Spirit
- Prov 25:28   It disciplines the body and mind
- Mt 6:33   It helps us set priorities in our life
- Mt 23:12   It humbles us before God
- Ps 63:1-2   It creates a longing for God

It is important to note, cleansing takes the good out with the bad. So with cleansing, more is not better. Pregnant, lactating women and children should never fast. If you have diabetes, hypoglycemia, or another chronic health problem, check with your doctor before starting a fast. Whenever you fast for more than three days, do so only under the supervision of a qualified health care professional. Remember, it took years to wear your body down, and it will take time to build it back up to its peak condition. Start fasting, but go slowly.

How to Fast

New Testament Christians practiced prayer and fasting regularly. Since there is no biblical command to fast, believers should be led by God through prayer concerning when and how often to fast. Below are some general guidelines.

- Fasting for twenty-four hours one day per month is a good practice for general health and will start you on a greater walk with our Lord.
- A one-day per week fast helps cleanse major organs, purifies your blood, and helps you lose excess weight

and helps strengthens your obedience to biblical principals.

- A three-day fast helps the body rid itself of toxins, cleanses the blood, and allows focused time for specific prayer needs.
- A five-day fast begins the process of healing, rebuilds the immune system, and can be used for intercessory prayer for family and friends.
- A ten-day fast can take care of many problems before they arise, may help fight illness, and gives way to greater awareness of God in your life and the world around you.

Types of fasts:

- Juice Fast—drink at least 80 oz. of distilled or reverse osmosis water and pure juices per day. Herbal and green teas also may be added. The best juice is lemon (juice of one lemon in one cup warm water with teaspoon of real grade B natural maple syrup), apple, beet, cabbage, carrot, celery, grape, or green drinks made with leafy green vegetables containing no sweeteners or additives. If you have to eat something, eat watermelon.
- Apple Fast—Eat three to four organically grown apples each day. Drink 64 oz. of reverse osmosis or distilled water and pure apple juice, with no sweeteners or additives, each day. Unsweetened herbal teas or green tea may also be added.
- Ease back into regular food slowly with salads and brown rice.

Important Tips

- Check with your doctor to make sure you are able to fast. People who are diabetic or with chronic health problems may not be able to fast.
- Use meal times as quite times with God.
- Keep a journal for Bible verses you have read and insights from devotionals used during the fast.
- When fasting, you may not be getting enough salt. If you feel lightheaded or dizzy, add a little sea salt to your drinks.
- Do not fast on water alone. It releases toxins too quickly, causing headaches.
- During your fast, be sure to get adequate rest.
- As toxins are being released from your body, you may experience fatigue, body odor, dry skin, skin eruptions, headaches, dizziness, irritability, anxiety, coughing, dark urine, dark smelly stools, or body aches. These symptoms are not serious and should pass quickly. To alleviate symptoms, drink herbal teas, such as peppermint, chamomile, or dandelion, during the fast.
- Continue your normal daily routine, except avoid strenuous exercise.
- Do not take fiber or unnecessary supplements during fasting; however, do continue any medications prescribed by your medical doctor.
- You should not drink coffee during your fast but can substitute with green tea.

Option to Fasting

Liver Cleanse without fasting – use the following recipe to cleanse without fasting.

Drink on an empty stomach first thing in the morning for 1 to 3 days.

- 1 cup organic fruit juice; apple or cranberry works best
- 2 lemons – fresh squeezed
- 1 cup distilled or spring water
- 1 TB virgin olive oil
- 1 clove garlic
- ½" fresh ginger root
- Crush garlic. Put all ingredients into blender.

Avoid coffee & alcohol during cleanse

Why do a Liver cleanse?

On a daily basis we ingest a heavy dose of unhealthy chemicals, toxins, preservatives, metals, antibiotics, hormones, genetically modified organisms, and other harmful substances from our air, food, and water supply. One of the many responsibilities of the liver is to remove these toxins and dangerous substances from the body. It does this by producing bile that binds these poisons and removes them safely. When the liver becomes overloaded by too many toxins, its function can become impaired. Since the liver is the largest and one of the most vital organs in the body, a damaged liver can result in serious disease and even death.

Step 4

Directly Supporting Health

Direct Support for a Healthy Lifestyle

> We remember the fish, which we did eat
> in Egypt freely; the cucumbers, and the
> melons and the leeks: and the onions, and
> the garlic.
>
> —Numbers 11:5

Cancer prevention is action taken to lower the chance of getting cancer. This year, about 1.6 million people will be diagnosed with cancer in the United States. Not only will this cause physical problems, it will hugely impact the patients and their families with the emotional distress caused by the cancer and the high costs of care. Over $100 billion has been spent on research, and $125 billion is spent on cancer care annually.

The majority of cancers are caused by lifestyle choices we make, the foods we eat, and our physical activity levels. Now is the time to take charge of your health.

Here are the basics:

- Allow yourself time for rest and relaxation.
- Avoid environmental toxins.
- Build your immune system with supplements and herbs.
- Do not worry.
- Exercise.
- Fast regularly.
- Give God time each day.
- If you choose to drink alcohol, do so only in moderation.
- Maintain a healthy weight.
- Make smart nutrition choices.
- Monitor your body for any changes that should be brought to the attention of medical professionals.
- Protect yourself from extended sun exposure.
- See a doctor regularly for checkups and health screenings.
- Stop smoking.

Start cancer prevention with the following thirty tips, one for each day of the month.

1. Spice up your food with cardamom, cayenne pepper, ginger, rosemary, sage, thyme, and turmeric.
2. Eat ten raw almonds a day—they contain laetrile, which may have anticancer properties and are a great source of essential fatty acids.

3. Put zest into your food with lots of garlic; research suggests it is linked to the prevention of cancers of the digestive system, especially esophageal, stomach and colon.

4. Drink three glasses of green tea each day—it's loaded with antioxidants found to inhibit cancer cells.

5. Smile till your face hurts.

6. Eat tomatoes—they contain lycopene, which may cut the risk of cervical, lung, stomach, and prostate cancers.

7. Be a prayer warrior and pray for someone new each day.

8. Enjoy tart cherries—they contain anthocyanins and antioxidants.

9. Find and use cleaning supplies with all natural ingredients.

10. Eat at least seven servings of fruits and vegetables every day.

11. Exercise regularly; it promotes oxygenation of the tissues.

12. Take a break from white foods—no white flour, sugar, potatoes, rice.

13. Limit your luncheon meats, hot dogs, or smoked or cured meats.

14. Filter your drinking water.

15. Stop topping your tank, continuing after the nozzle clicks interferes with the vapor recovery system that keeps cancer-causing chemicals out of the air.

16. Keep an eye on the grill when cooking meat; charred, well-done meats contain cancer-causing heterocyclic amines.

17. Drink at least eight cups of water a day; this dilutes the concentration of cancer-causing agents and flushes them out of our body.

18. Choose the darkest varieties of vegetables for your salad; they contain more antioxidants.

19. Snack on Brazil nuts; they are loaded with selenium, which may lower the risk of bladder, lung, or colorectal cancer.

20. Walk briskly two hours per week; it cuts the risk of breast cancer by 18 percent.

21. Wear blue or red clothes to protect against the sun's UV rays.

22. Choose dark chocolate—1.5 ounces of 70 percent cocoa is divine and an anticancer food.

23. Wash your fresh fruits and vegetables before eating to remove pesticides.

24. Choose meat free of antibiotics and added hormones.

25. Adding more calcium to your diet may help reduce the chance for colon cancer.

26. Drop ten pounds—being overweight accounts for 20 percent of all cancer deaths among women and 14 percent among men

27. Sit at least eight feet away from television sets to avoid low-level radiation leakage.

28. Use extra virgin olive oil; it contains antioxidants that have been linked with the slower progression of cancer.

29. Try stone fruit—peaches, plums, and nectarines have demonstrated efficacy against breast cancer cells in lab tests.

30. Cancer hates cabbage—enjoy vegetables from the cabbage family, which includes cabbage, broccoli, cauliflower, Brussels sprouts, collard greens, and kale.

Herbs

Better is a dinner of herbs where love is,
than a fatted ox with hatred.

—Proverbs 15:16

According to the World Health Organization[17], cancer incidences have steadily increased at an alarming rate. Take away the major culprits like smoking, genetic risks, poor diet, stress, and lack of exercise, and we're still left with lots of disease. The rise in cancer may be due to replacing the high diversity, high fiber, high antioxidant, low cholesterol, holistic lifestyle of our ancestors with the current sedentary, high fat, highly refined sugar and flour lifestyle. Natural antibiotics from herbs such as garlic and olive leaf, both used in biblical times, are less a part of diets today. Billions of dollars are spent on the latest and greatest silver bullets that are loaded with side effects and taken off the market within ten years. It makes more sense to emphasize the natural,

---

[17] Bosely Sarah, "Cancer cases expected to increase 70% over next 20 years", The Guardian, posted Feb 03, 2014, http://www.theguardian.com/society/2014/feb/03/worldwide-cancer-cases-soar-next-20-years.

preventative healing properties of plants that USDA research has confirmed: aloes to treat radiation burns, chicory for HIV, cinnamon for diabetes, dill for colic, benzaldehyde from figs for cancer, garlic for hypertension, scopolamine from mandrakes for vertigo, choline from nettles to prevent Alzheimer's, oregano to prevent cataracts, turmeric for lymphoma, and walnuts to lower cholesterol levels. Combine the potential of herbs with the advances in modern Western medicine and we could experience a healthier future.

As a naturopath, I am always amazed at the many ways herbs can be used to assist with our health. Proven through thousands of years, their effectiveness has been a flagship for natural health. Below are some plants to build a powerful army of cancer-fighting warriors from biblical times.

Aloe

From biblical times to the present, aloes have been a giant among herbs and herbal medicine. Nicodemus brought a mixture of myrrh and aloes to wash the crucified body of Christ. Setting sail for the new world, Christopher Columbus wrote in his diary, "All is well. Aloe is on board." Used to treat burns, scrapes, scratches, and bites, aloe also aids healing. It exhibits anesthetic and antibacterial action and increases blood and lymph flow in the area of damage. The root decoction has been used for stomach cancer and as an aloe poultice for tumors.

Alliums—Garlic

Garlic has served as a medicinal aid for nearly five thousand years. Roman soldiers ate a daily ration of garlic to sustain them on long marches. The ancient Egyptian pyramid builders also ate garlic daily for strength and stamina. Hippocrates, the father of medicine, used garlic for everything from infections to intestinal disorders. Allicin, a powerful antibiotic found in garlic, protects the body from carcinogens and bacteria, and facilitates healing. Colon, brain, lung, prostate, kidney, and breast cancers all react to garlic, which appears to help kill the cells and shrink tumors.

Dandelion Root

A bitter herb like chicory of the Bible, both are cultivated for the medicinal qualities of their roots and as a coffee substitute. Dandelion is considered by many to be one of the bitter herbs of Passover. Researchers in Windsor found that an extract from dandelion root caused cancer cells to commit suicide (apoptosis) without harming non-cancerous cells. The dandelion root (not the leaf, which is a fabulous diuretic) appears to disable the cancerous cells of leukemia and a variety of other types of cancer, including bone cancer, pancreatic cancer, colon cancer, and neuroblastoma. Additionally, dandelions are known to be high in antioxidants and great for improving liver function. Clearly, drinking dandelion tea could help prevent cancer. And since there is no known toxicity to humans in consuming dandelions, it's probably a good idea to make dandelion tea a part of your daily routine. Pour one cup of boiling water over chopped dandelion root and let steep ten minutes. Add a little green tea to add flavor and double the power of the drink against cancer.

Dill

"For dill is not threshed with a threshing sledge, nor is the cartwheel driven over cumin, but dill is beaten out with a rod and cumin with a club" (Isaiah 27:27). It was so important in biblical times that records indicate that the seeds, stems, and leaves were subject to being tithed. Dill contains compounds that are beneficial for fighting cancer. Called *monoterpenes*, these compounds stimulate an enzyme, glutathione-S-transferase. This enzyme is a powerful antioxidant that is particularly effective at targeting different types of carcinogens, especially free radicals. Dill also contains essential oils, which are known to stimulate digestive juices, activating bile production helping the intestines function healthily.

Figs

The fig tree is first mentioned in the Bible with Adam and Eve sewing fig leaves together for clothes. In biblical imagery, the fig tree symbolizes prosperity and peace. It was one of the seven plants God promised the Hebrews when they reached the Promised Land. Medicinally, figs may hold the cures for cancer, AIDS, and diabetes. Hezekiah was dying from a malignant tumor. The prophet Isaiah pounded the fruit into pulp for a poultice and applied it to the tumor. Thus with God's power, he healed Hezekiah's malignancy. Figs contain psoralen, an antidote to Staphylococcus. An active ingredient in figs, benzaldehyde has been effective in experiments on mice afflicted with carcinoma. It has been used to treat cancers of the gums, neck, liver, uterus, and testicles.

Flax

Linen from flax is one of the world's oldest fabrics. Israelite priests wore linen garments. Flaxseed oil was used in the embalming process. The three principal components of flax are alpha-linolenic acid (ALA), dietary fiber, and polyphenolics (lignans). ALA has been shown to prevent inflammation, retard tumor growth, as well as boost the immune system. The lignans in flaxseed are particularly useful in preventing breast and colon cancers. Use ground flax seed daily in your diet as an additional source of fiber, an omega-3 essential fatty acid, and to prevent cancer.

Olive

The olive tree has been cultivated for more than six thousand years. Jesus spent the night before his capture and eventual crucifixion in the Garden of Gethsemane, which means "the garden with the olive press." Olive oil—and specifically its oleuropein content—is the key component of the Mediterranean diet's anti-cancer effects. Studies show that oleuropein's antioxidant effects help it battle cancer formation at its earliest stages. Olive leaf extracts inhibit DNA damage, which is the very first step in the development of malignant cells. Olive leaf compounds are known to inhibit growth factors and disrupt signaling pathways. Oleuropein also suppresses an enzyme cancer cells rely on to derive and store energy from its main source of fuel, carbohydrates.

Turmeric

It's not known for sure, but many herbalist believe turmeric could have been the saffron mentioned in Song of Solomon 4:14. Turmeric is the yellow powder that gives curry its color and plays a huge role in Ayurveda medicine. Indians have a lower percentage of cancers than Americans, and this has inspired studies across the globe. Studies by Dr. Goel at Baylor University Medical Center[18] have found the active ingredient, curcumin, has killed different types of cancer cells without the toxic side of traditional therapies. The spice is absorbed into the blood stream and flows to all the organs in the body, so it also reduces the spreading of the disease.

Many herbs appear to seek and destroy specific forms of cancer. Research with many herbs has shown a lot of promise. Additionally, dietary and nutritional factors have been studied, which may help prevent certain cancers.

---

[18]   Nick Tate, "Common Spice That Treats Cancer", Newsmax. com, updated May 30 2014, http://www.newsmax.com/health/ health-news/curcumin-cancer.

According to the American Cancer Society, [19]one-third of cancers can be attributed to dietary factors. If you are concerned about the possibility of developing a certain kind of cancer, consider the following recommendation for prevention.

Bladder Cancer

Cruciferous vegetables have been credited with lowering the risk of bladder cancer due to their antioxidant and other cancer-fighting compounds. Cruciferous vegetables include broccoli, Brussels sprouts, cabbage, cauliflower, and kale. Drinking a lot of water helps to dilute carcinogens and increase urination, lessening the time any carcinogens in the bladder have to do any damage. Taking vitamins A (beta-carotene), C, and E may also help.

Breast Cancer

Green tea contains catechins and flavonoids, which may be protective against estrogen-dominant breast cancer. Eat a high-fiber diet based on fresh fruits and vegetables. Fiber keeps toxic wastes from being absorbed into the bloodstream. A great fiber is ground flax seeds, which also contain lignins and omega-3 essential fatty acids; both are known to reduce breast cancer risk. Limit carbohydrates;

---

[19] "Family Cancer Syndromes", American Cancer Society, accessed March 23, 2015, http://cancer.org/cancer/cancercauses/genetics and cancer

studies show that women who ate the most carbs were twice as likely to have breast cancer.

Cervical Cancer

A diet low in fatty meats, such as cold cuts, red meat, cheeses, and white bread, and high in soy products, fruits, dark green vegetables, tomatoes, whole grains, and yogurt are the best protection. Folic acid, B9, not only aids in prevention but has also been known to reverse precancerous changes in cervical cells.

Colorectal Cancer

A vegetarian diet or a diet low in red meat with lots of fruits and vegetables offers the best protection. Studies show that aged garlic slows the rate of progression of established colon cancer cells. Coffee in moderation has also been shown to reduce colon cancer risk. Calcium, beta-carotene, selenium and vitamins C and E have been linked to reduced risk of colon cancer. Probiotics may also inhibit colon cancer.

Esophageal Cancer

A diet high in fruits (especially tomatoes) and vegetables is important to prevent this type of cancer. Adding foods containing omega-3 essential fatty acids, vitamins A and C, as well as vitamin B2, riboflavin, is also critical. Green tea contains catechins, which are known to inhibit esophageal cancer. Avoid salty, pickled, or moldy foods (like cheese).

Leukemia

Plenty of fluids, blood-cleansing herbs like burdock or butcher's broom, and immune-building fruits and vegetables are important to prevent Leukemia. Soy products may offer protection against leukemia. Numerous studies have found the bioflavonoid quercetin to have anti-leukemia properties.

Lymphoma

Keeping the body moving on a regular basis to cleanse the lymph as well as eating a diet high in fiber is critical to prevent lymphoma cancers. A diet with low- glycemic foods and loaded with vegetables is important.

Prostate Cancer

Maintain a whole foods diet—no processed food. Green tea and lycopene (tomatoes, watermelon are a good sources) may prevent tumor growth. Include foods that are high in zinc, like pumpkin seeds, spinach, and sunflower seeds. Drink half your body weight in ounces of water each day (100 lbs would drink 50 oz/day) to keep the prostate working efficiently. Restrict diary products and red meat. Saw palmetto not only helps with enlarged prostate but will also help fight cancer development.

Skin Cancer

Eat a diet that is high in antioxidants, including orange foods and cruciferous vegetables. Drink four cups of green tea daily for prevention. Alfalfa, burdock, dandelion, marshmallow root, and oat straw keep the skin healthy and enhance tissue repair.

Stomach Cancer

Broccoli, onions, garlic, and pineapple are high in sulfur and offer protection against stomach cancer. A tablespoon of coconut oil will also help heal stomach tissue and discourage development of cancer cells. Antioxidants from fruits and vegetables are the best sources of protection.

Step 5

Evaluate Your Health Regularly

Evaluation

Take charge of your body. Stay on the offensive. Make it a priority to have an annual checkup with routine blood work. Have regular cancer screening tests and checkups.

Regular self-exams can increase your chances of discovering cancer early when treatment is most likely to be successful.

The American Cancer Society recommends the following screening guidelines for most adults.

Breast cancer

- Yearly mammograms are recommended starting at age forty and continuing for as long as a woman is in good health
- Breast self-exam is an option for women starting in their twenties.

Some women—because of their family history, a genetic tendency, or certain other factors—should be screened with MRI in addition to mammograms. (The number of women who fall into this category is small: less than 2 percent of all the women in the United States.) Talk with your doctor about your history and whether you should have additional tests at an earlier age.

Colorectal cancer and polyps

Beginning at age fifty, both men and women should follow one of these testing schedules:

Tests that primarily find cancer

- Yearly fecal occult blood test
- Yearly fecal immunochemical test
- Stool DNA test

Talk to your doctor about which test is best for you.

Cervical cancer

- Cervical cancer screening (testing) should begin at age twenty-one.
- Women between ages twenty-one and sixty-five should have a Pap test every three years.
- Women over age sixty-five who have had regular cervical cancer testing with normal results should not be tested for cervical cancer

Some women, because of their health history, may need to have a different screening schedule for cervical cancer. Talk to your doctor or nurse about your history.

Lung cancer

If you meet all of the following criteria, then you might be a candidate for screening:

- Fifty-five to seventy-four years of age
- In fairly good health
- Have at least a thirty-pack-per-year smoking history *and* are either still smoking or have quit smoking within the last fifteen years

Prostate cancer

The American Cancer Society recommends that men make an informed decision with their doctor about whether to be tested for prostate cancer.

Bibliography

Scripture taken from The Holy Bible, New International Version. Copyright 1973, 1978,1984 by International Bible Society. Used by permission of Zondervan, Grand Rapids, MI. All rights reserved.

"Soda Studies", Beverage Digest, accessed Mar 23, 2015, http://www.beveragelife.ru/beverage-industry-statistics/sodas-studies/.

Bosely Sarah, "Cancer cases expected to increase 70% over next 20 years", The Guardian, posted Feb 03, 2014, http://www.theguardian.com/society/2014/feb/03/worldwide-cancer-cases-soar-next-20-years.[20]

Balch, Phyllis A, CNC, *Prescription for Nutritional Healing: A Practical A-to-Z Reference to Drug-Free Remedies Using Vitamins, Minerals, Herbs & Food Supplements.* 5th ed. New York: Avery, 2010.

Beliveau, Richard PhD, and Denis Gingras PhD, *Foods to Fight Cancer: Essential foods to help prevent cancer.* New York: DK Publishing, 2007.

Bernaardi, L. P. Sleight, G. Bandinelli, et al, "Effect of Rosary Prayer and Yoga Mantras on Autonomic Cardiovascular Rhythms", British Medical Journal 323 (2001): 1446-49 and Thayer, J. F. and E. Sternberg, "Beyond Heart Rate Variability: Vagal Regulation of Allostatic Systems", Annuals of the New York Academy of Sciences 1008 (2006): 361-72.

"Cancer costs projected to reach at least $158 billion in 2020", National Institutes of Health, accessed March 23, 2015, http://www.cancer.gov/newscenter/newsfrom nci/2011/costcancer

Duke, James A, *Herbs of the Bible: 2000 years of plant medicine.* 2nd ed. Warsaw IN: Whitman Publications. 2007

Easley, Thomas, AHG and Steven Horne, AHG, *Modern Herbal Medicine.* UT: School of Modern Herbal Medicine. 2014

"Family Cancer Syndromes", American Cancer Society, accessed March 23, 2015, http://cancer.org/cancer/ cancercauses/genetics and cancer

Frahm, Dave, *A Cancer Battle Plan Sourcebook.* NY: Jeremy P Tarcher/Putnam. 2000

Horne, Steven H, AHG, *Nature's Pharmacy An Essential Materia Medica of Modern American Herbalism*. St. George, UT: Tree of Light Publishing. 2007

"Importance of Sleep: Six reasons not to scrimp on sleep", Harvard Health Publications, modified Jan 1, 2006\ http://health.harvard.edu/press_releases/importance of sleep.

Meares, Ainslie, MDDPM, "Regression of Osteogenic Sarcoma metastases associated with intensive mediation," Medical Journal of Australia 2, no.9 (1978): 433.

Loecher, Barbara, "Slash Your Cancer Risk", *Prevention Magazine*, November 3, 2011.

"Positive thinking: stop negative self-talk to reduce stress", Mayo Clinic, accessed March 23, 2015, http://mayoclinic.org/healthy-lviing/stress-management.

Servan-Schreiber, David, MD, PhD, *Anti Cancer: A New Way of Life*, New York: Penguin Group Inc. 2009

Shaw, Jerry, "Health Benefits of Positive Thinking", Livestrong.com, last updated Jan 28,2015, http://livestrong.com/article/75627-health-benefits-positive-thinking/.

Tate, Nick, "Common Spice That Treats Cancer", Newsmax.com, updated May 30 2014, http://www.newsmax.com/health/health-news/curcumin-cancer.

The Congressional Prevention Coalition, "Stress Prevention". Institute of Science, Technology and Public Policy, Presented June 24, 1998, http://istpp.org/coalition/stress_prevention.html

Tozer A. W., "Created To Worship God", WordPress.com, updated Dec 1, 2011, https://psalm86nine.wordpress.com/2011/12/01.quote-from-tozer

Visintainer, M.A., JR. Volpicelli and M.C. P. Seligman, "Tumor Rejection in Rats After Inescapable or Escapable Shock," Science 216 (1982): 437-39.

Young-Chou, Lee, "Heme Oxygenase-1: emerging target of cancer therapy". Journal of Biomedical Science 22 (2015): accessed March 21, 2015, doi:1186/s12929-015-0128-0.

Printed in the United States
By Bookmasters